5-MINUTE FII

D0829616

relieve
stress

20 QUICK TECHNIQUES

KATRIN SCHUBERT, MD

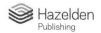

Hazelden
Publishing

Hazelden Publishing
Center City, Minnesota 55012
hazelden.org/bookstore

ISBN: 978-1-61649-638-8

Library of Congress Cataloging-in-Publication Data is on file
with the Library of Congress.

Editor's notes
The names, details, and circumstances may have been changed to
protect the privacy of those mentioned in this publication.

Any information in this book is offered for your well-being
only and is not intended to diagnose illness, nor is it a substitute
for medical care. Please contact your physician or hospital for any
health care concerns.

Do not use these techniques while driving a car or operating
heavy machinery.

20 19 18 17 16   1 2 3 4 5 6

Cover design: Kathi Dunn, Dunn + Associates
Interior illustrations: David Spohn
Author photo: Deb Stagg
Developmental editor: Sid Farrar
Production editor: Heather Silsbee

With gratitude to Lyell and Jillian, my family,
friends, and my clients
who have taught me everything!
And to Thomas for his invaluable support.

CONTENTS

Introduction

The inspiration for this book came from many years working as a holistic medical doctor outside of the allopathic (traditional Western) medical approach. I am licensed as a physician in Germany. I work and live in Canada and have been in private holistic health care for over two decades. While practicing in the 1990s, I observed that my patients' lives were increasingly burdened with layoffs, cutbacks, and double-income earners needing to work overtime just to make ends meet.

From the vantage point of the second decade of the twenty-first century, the nineties now look like a still life of serenity. Today, traffic, climate change, and electromagnetic pollution are compromising our health and well-being. Instead of visiting with friends in person, we now spend hours tapping on our electronic devices, opting to interact in virtual reality, which damages our quality of life and weakens our immune system. My colleagues and I began to notice that, in contrast to the run-of-the-mill health concerns of a decade ago, our practices were becoming flooded with people suffering from ever-increasing and often debilitating anxiety and stress.

My clientele also shifted from mainly women with emotional concerns to include men and adolescents complaining about high levels of fear and nervousness. Men were no longer able to suppress their anxieties the way they had been brought up to do. And many young people were unable to deal with life due to depression and fear of the future.

Curious about this phenomenon, I started searching for answers. The underlying causes of increased stress are countless. Environmental toxins, substance misuse, shifting values, reduced time off from work, social and family time constraints, and fear of financial instability are but a few.

The good news is that there is much we can do by ourselves, for ourselves. We have tools we can apply effectively to help us cope with the stress of everyday life.

Relief from the Mental Race

We are told that all power lies in the present moment. Yet, unlike other animals, humans find it challenging to stay focused in the present. Excessive worry means we spend too much time thinking of the future, while dwelling on the past can lock us in anger, sadness, and fear.

Do you spend some or even many of your precious days feeling rattled? Does the swirl of sudden bad news unhinge your mind and body? Do people challenge you, pushing sensitive buttons and making you feel angry or anxious, triggering a reminder of some past painful event that awakens difficult emotions? Does it seem that at times your whole being is struggling to find the ground under your feet, that you are sinking into the quicksand of negativity? Then you are just like me, part of the human race In our Western world of timelines, social frameworks, and family and work dynamics that have a mind of their own.

Being stuck in acute anxiety or negative thoughts robs us of life's pleasures and can even make us sick. Research has shown what we intuitively know:

a challenged mind and trapped emotions can cause physical illness.

In part 1 of this book, you'll find twenty proven techniques—including acupressure, visualization, and affirmations—that you can apply in five minutes or less to relieve stress and anxiety in everyday life, wherever you are. You already have all you need within you: no gadgets, extra expenses, batteries, or matching power cords are required! In part 2, you'll find background and theoretical information on the techniques to help you understand how and why they work.

No single intervention, including those in this book, will solve all of the complex personal and societal problems that cause mental unrest. But regardless of your age or background, the techniques I have gathered can give you temporary relief from the stress caused by the mental-race-with-no-end we find ourselves in. They can reset the thermostat of your nervous system and bring calmness that results in mental, emotional, and physical well-being to see you through difficult situations.

I invite you to try out these techniques and hope that you will find several that make your life calmer and more manageable.

Enjoy the journey!

. . .

Publisher's note:
Stress is a major contributor to cravings for unhealthy foods, alcohol, and other substances and a few of the techniques in this book are also recommended in another 5-Minute First Aid for the Mind title, *Reduce Craving.*

Part I:

The Techniques

RACHEL WAS A SIXTEEN-YEAR-OLD STUDENT with special needs. When Rachel was in her mid-teens, she was functioning on the level of an eleven-year-old. Intellectually younger all her life, she had suffered from anxiety that was even greater than what is normally experienced by many teens, causing her to feel overwhelmed much of the time.

Rachel was asked to move to a different classroom, and while adjusting to her new surroundings she decided to teach her classmates and new teacher several exercises she had learned from her previous teacher. Those exercises, which are the techniques presented in this book, had improved her coping skills and lessened her anxiety, and she was hopeful that her new classmates would benefit from them as much as she had.

In that spirit I share these techniques with you and hope that by using them you find more peace of mind, as Rachel and her classmates did.

TECHNIQUE 1

Square Breathing

Lucia was sitting in the waiting area of her doctor's office. Two weeks earlier, she had found a lump in her breast and was now waiting to hear the results of her medical test. She was terrified. For the past few weeks her mind had been cycling through the same thoughts like a spinning top, leaving her unable to focus and trapped in fear. Her breath was shallow and she felt a nervous sweat breaking out over her body. She was afraid she was going to faint.

Applying square breathing by using a table top in the waiting room turned out to be the perfect technique to help Lucia calm her mind.

•

Julie used this technique to slow down her "busy mind." Here is how she described the results:

When my mind is busy with the ten thousand "things" in my life—the calls I have to make, the bills that need to be paid, the tires that need rotating, the cat that needs to see the vet, my child who needs help—I have trouble falling asleep no matter how tired I am.

I start "breathing the square," and when I closely pay attention to my eye movements and align them with my breath, my busy thoughts vanish. It feels as if my brain is taking a deep breath because it gets a break from working so hard on all my thoughts.

✳

Brad tried the technique for insomnia. He often had trouble sleeping and woke up with thoughts crowding his mind. He reported that square breathing took his mind off his thoughts, and the next thing he remembered was waking up in the morning.

HOW TO DO IT

Find a square or rectangular object in your surroundings. It can be a picture frame or door if you are indoors, or a car window, section of a sidewalk, or flower box if you are out in the city. Even the great outdoors will offer squares or rectangles in the form of stones, bushes, or fences.

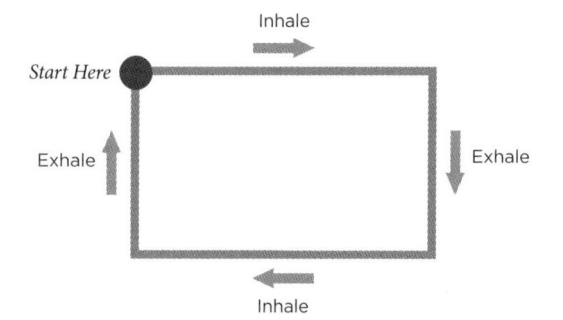

Now move your eyes from the top left corner of your box horizontally to the right side while inhaling. This means you move in a clockwise fashion. Be mindful to slow down your eye movements and breath. Once you reach the upper right corner, move your eyes downward in a very deliberate fashion while slowly exhaling. Breathe in along the bottom corner from right to left, and then breathe out from the bottom left upward to your starting point. Keep moving your eyes along the square while slowing down your breath, inhaling along the top and bottom edges and exhaling along the sides. Ideally your out-breath should last as long as your in-breath. Breathe around the square for several rounds or two to five minutes, and repeat the exercise if you feel your uneasy thoughts returning. You may also want to change the direction of your eye movement to counterclockwise for added benefit.

You may notice that your mind becomes occupied with moving your eyes from one corner to the next while synchronizing your breathing, leaving no "mind space" for anxious thoughts. You may feel a sense of calm, and it can help reset your nervous system. (This technique is also included in my book *Reduce Craving: 20 Quick Techniques*.)

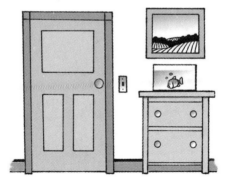

Find a square or rectangular object in your surroundings.

TECHNIQUE 2

Polka-Dot Picture
FINDING THE RIGHT PERSPECTIVE

Suzanne felt the floor drop beneath her when she found out that her sixteen-year-old daughter was pregnant. It felt as if her world were coming apart as the impending problems of her daughter's teenage motherhood loomed like a mountain in front of her. Her dreams for her daughter's future seemed to shatter.

The Polka-Dot Picture helped Suzanne put the issue into a broader context, enabling her to cope better.

HOW IT WORKS

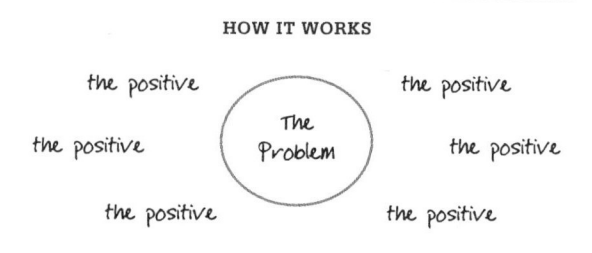

Write a problem in the center of a circle and positive facts that put the problem in a better perspective around the circle.

Get a piece of paper and a pen or pencil. Draw a small circle in the center of the paper and write the problem that is occupying your mind in the center of the circle. Now focus on the space outside this circle and start writing all the positive aspects of the situation that you can think of.

Here is an example:

Center circle:
My teenage daughter is pregnant.

Outside area:
She is healthy; she will be able to finish her education; excellent/good/sufficient medical care is available to her; I have experience in raising a child and can be of help; there are support staff and support groups available; there are many others in the same situation; she will be able to care for her child; she will gain valuable experience; she will be able to live a full life; a child is a joyful addition to one's life.

And here is what it looks like on paper:

SUZANNE'S EXAMPLE

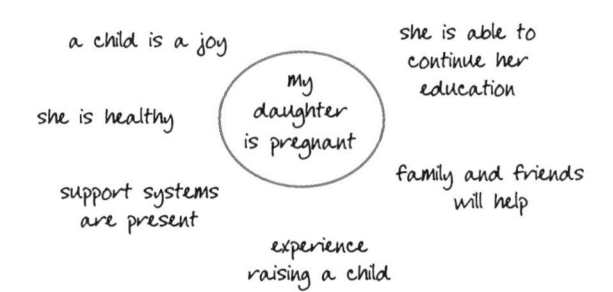

16

TECHNIQUE 3

"Happy Point" Acupressure

Desiree woke up in the morning feeling under the weather. There was a sensation of pressure around her eyes and sinuses, and she felt rather low and a bit confused. Her mood was "off"; maybe she was getting a cold, as she had been around people with the sniffles.

Despite not feeling well she had to get out of bed, put on a smile, and "connect her brain cells," as she had to give an important presentation at work. Her boss relied on her and would be gauging her performance.

Massaging the acupressure point labeled Li4 on acupressure point charts, also called the "happy point," on both hands for about five minutes helped to clear her head, improve her mood, and perk her up enough to feel confident during her presentation.

Li4 (Large Intestine 4) is an acupressure point located in the fleshy, muscular part of the hand between the thumb and index finger. Acupressure on Li4 can ease headaches and cold symptoms, stimulate your immune system, and make you feel happier.

You may notice that this area feels tender or achy when you massage it. This is a good sign, and it means you should work it for several minutes. It is best to massage this area between your thumb and index finger from both sides, gently pinching the palm side and the back of your hand at the same time. Massage each hand for three to five minutes and repeat if you wish. Over time this acupressure point may become less tender, indicating that you are in better balance.

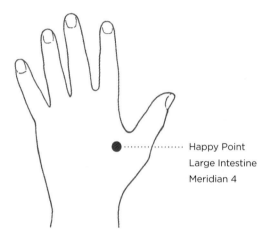

Happy Point
Large Intestine
Meridian 4

Massage each hand for three to five minutes.

TECHNIQUE 4

BodyTalk Cortices

Fifteen-year-old Cole could no longer contain his emotions. He felt overwhelmed, and he started to sob uncontrollably. First his grandfather, whom he had been very close to, had passed away, then his best friend from school had moved, and to top it off his parents had separated. His life had been turned upside down, and there was no silver lining to his cloud.

His father tried to console him by using the Cortices technique on him, which helped Cole to balance his brain, relax his breathing, and calm himself down. He was now able to talk and express his feelings.

•

Ashley had studied hard for the exam. Passing this test was very important to her. But as she sat in front of her test papers, she could barely remember what she had learned. Her head was swimming and her heart was racing with nervous anticipation. Her brain was unable to recall the information she knew she had memorized only the day before. The Cortices technique helped her to reconnect her brain pathways so she could retrieve the information she had learned.

•

Timothy is a professional actor and loves his work. Although performance rehearsals are very intense, just before the show begins he usually experiences joyful anticipation as the curtain rises. But there are moments before a show when Timothy's nerves would get frazzled, when he worried about his lines, who would be in the audience, and whether all would go smoothly. Timothy found the Cortices technique to be very centering and calming. When he did Cortices during rehearsals and before a show, he often noticed his mind became clearer and he regained his confidence.

•

The Cortices technique is part of the amazing BodyTalk system and BodyTalk Access developed by Dr. John Veltheim.

1st position

Hold with your left hand: Gently cup your left hand at the back of your head just above your hairline. Always keep half of your hand (your palm) on the left side of your head and the fingers on the right side. The crease between your palm and your fingers lies over the center part of the back of your head. Make sure you follow this pattern for all of the positions of your left hand.

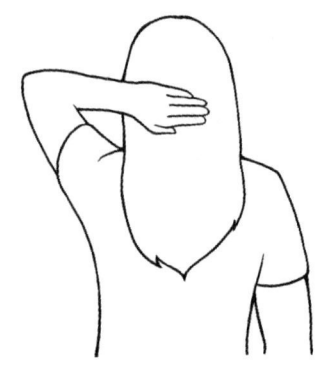

First hand position: bottom of the head where it meets the neck.

The tapping part of the technique will be repeated with every hand position.

Tapping Pattern

Tap with your right hand: Use your right hand to very gently tap on top of your head with your fingers spread to cover the midline and right and left sides of the top of your head. Do this for about one full breath cycle in and out.

Now move the same hand to the center of your chest bone and tap again for about one full breath in and out. It does not matter how often you tap; just be relaxed and gentle about it. You may choose to tap a little longer if you like.

Use just as much pressure as you would on a baby bird.

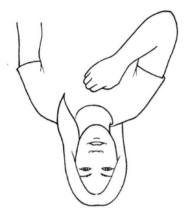

Tap the top of your head with right hand, fingers spread out.

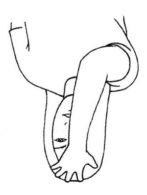

Tap middle of your chest with right hand.

2nd position

Hold with your left hand: Move your left hand just above position 1 to what we will call position 2. (You are going to systematically cover the whole head one hand-width at a time.)

Tap with your right hand: Follow the tapping pattern described on page 23.

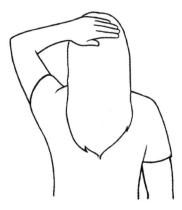

Second hand position on back of head.

3rd position

Hold with your left hand: Move your left hand up to the next position on the back of the top of your head (where one may wear a beanie or yarmulke).

Tap with your right hand: Follow the tapping pattern described on page 23. Your right hand will tap on top of your left hand in this step.

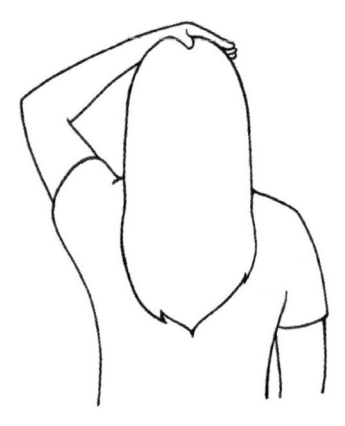

Third hand position on top of head.

4th position

Hold with your left hand: Cover your front hairline and forehead with your left hand from one side to the other.

Tap with your right hand: Follow the tapping pattern described on page 23. You may want to hold and tap for more than one breath in this position. If it feels soothing, hold and tap a while longer.

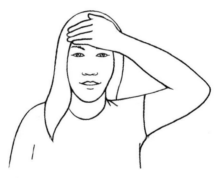

Fourth hand position on forehead.

5th position

Both hands: Place your hands on either side of your head just above your ears and gently hold this position for at least one breath cycle. Keeping your left hand in place above your left ear, tap with your right hand first on top of your head and then on your chest bone. Then put your right hand back above your right ear for a while longer.

This position helps your emotional brain and may feel very calming.

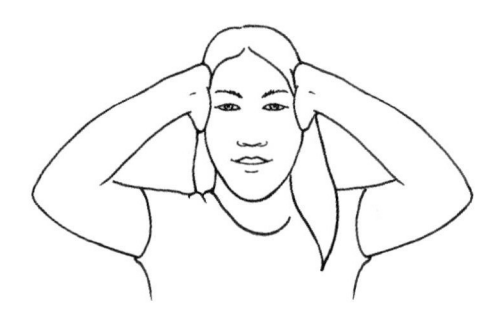

Fifth hand position with both hands above ears.

THE 5 HAND POSITIONS:

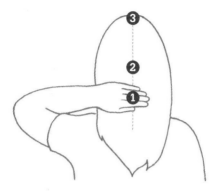

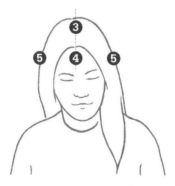

This Is What Is Happening

Bridging from one side of the head to the other side of the head with your hand helps your body to form a stronger energetic connection between the two sides of your brain. (One side of your brain is called a "cortex"; the two sides are called "cortices.") The two sides of the brain are connected by a path called the "corpus callosum" (CC) that acts like a superhighway. When this superhighway is open, information can flow freely. We then feel good, cope well, and remember things easily.

Under any kind of stress, the highway (the CC) gets blocked. Having a disconnect between the right (creative) and left (logical) sides of the brain can trigger stress, overwhelm you, and cause physical and emotional pain.

You may remember a time when you studied very hard but during the stress of the exam you could not retrieve the necessary information. Perhaps if you had done the Cortices technique your brain pathways would have energetically reconnected and your memory would have improved. The same is true for emotional upset or physical pain. The Cortices technique can reset your brain pathways, helping you feel better right away.

When we get injured our brain goes into shock, which slows down the healing process. In such instances, applying the Cortices technique right away can help to rebalance your nervous system. By resetting your brain, your healing process becomes more effective. If you are injured, you will probably have to repeat this technique several times. Hold the positions for a longer amount of time if desired. You can do Cortices as often as you feel the need to. Many people notice a sensation of well-being in their body and mind after using this technique.

TECHNIQUE 5

I Am All Ear

THE MIRACLE OF THE AURICLE

Did you know that the "auricle," or external portion of the ear, represents every part of the body? In addition to the classical Chinese way of understanding acupuncture and acupressure, science has discovered that acupuncture and acupressure on certain body parts, called "reflex organs," can effectively treat the entire body and mind. The ear is such a reflex organ. By massaging certain spots on your ear, you can ease your mind and help your body heal. The brilliant French doctor Paul Nogier discovered this phenomenon, and it changed the world of acupuncture! Dr. Nogier developed the sophisticated modality of ear acupuncture as both a diagnostic and treatment tool.

As an instructor of the BodyTalk system from which the Cortices technique is taken, I teach long days. Students need to take in volumes of material within a short time while simultaneously understanding how to apply this new way of healing. After a couple days of classes students feel mentally tired, and this simple ear massage technique helps to refresh their brains.

An energetic massage of your ear can restore your fatigued mind and body and enhance memory recall. Stimulating certain areas on the ear can also help relieve depression and calm you down when you are irritated.

HOW TO DO IT

Lightly pinch your ears between your index finger and your thumb. Move along the outside of your ears from the bottom to the top, rubbing and massaging them. You will notice that there are tender and sometimes exquisitely achy spots. Pay extra attention to those areas and work them a little longer and harder. You want to feel "good" pain but avoid intense or sharp pain. By doing this you have just given your spine a massage, and you may already feel a little more invigorated.

Now move to your earlobe. The science of auricular acupressure reveals that your earlobe represents your brain, face, jaw, neurotransmitters, and emotions.

On the outer part of your earlobe you will find a point that lifts your spirits.

Now massage your earlobes really well, and *voila!* — you just invigorated your brain and face. Most people feel more alive, more awake, and more ready to face their tasks and the world around them after they have performed this technique.

EAR MASSAGE POINTS

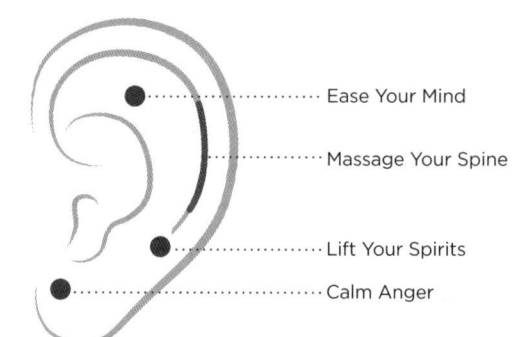

Ease Your Mind

Massage Your Spine

Lift Your Spirits

Calm Anger

You can repeat this massage anytime you're upset and stressed out, no matter where you are. (A modified version of this technique is also included in my book *Reduce Craving: 20 Quick Techniques*.)

The Grief
(Anger, Fear, or Other Upset)
Box

Four-year-old Katie was very upset. Her parents had separated a couple of years earlier, and her father, whom she missed very much, had forgotten her birthday. She went to her mother and told her with a trembling voice that her heart was "achy." Her mom took Katie to her room and found a treasure box on Katie's shelf right beside her favorite stuffed ostrich. Her mother helped her to use the box to "siphon off" some of her grief for safekeeping, and it made Katie feel much lighter.

HOW TO DO IT

Pick a special box or other container that you may have around your home, school, or place of work. It can be a wooden box, a woven basket, a bucket, or even an envelope or brown paper bag.

Pay attention to your body and notice where you might be feeling tension, pain, or other discomfort. Now imagine collecting this grief, anger, fear, or other upset in your hands from any of those places in your body that you feel are holding it and put that upset in your container of choice. It might help to write the particular feeling on a slip of paper and put that in the container as well. Leave it there for safekeeping—you will be able to get back to it for more processing when your feelings have settled, even if that doesn't happen for quite a while. Remember that you can add to your box at any time.

Placing these feelings in your Grief Box can make your body-mind feel lighter for the moment without suppressing or denying the emotion.

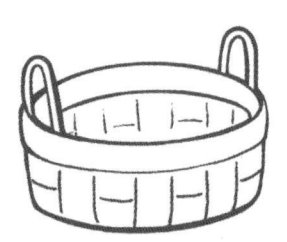

TECHNIQUE 7

Healthy Thought Exchange

There are times when I am preoccupied with judging and criticizing situations and people—including myself—which makes my life more stressful. My mind dwells on what went wrong and what I should or shouldn't have done, playing a series of "what ifs" like a broken record. Usually it takes a while for my conscious mind to notice the internal negative dialogue running in the background. When I become aware of my negative thinking, I employ the following technique that Ruth, one of my great healer friends and mentors, taught me.

•

HOW TO DO IT

Read this affirmation aloud or silently to yourself. After a while you may be able to remember it by heart and use this technique any place you are. You may need to repeat this affirmation several times before you notice the shift to healthier, happier, and more productive thinking.

From the power of the creation within me,
From the essence of all that I am,
I let go of all energies within and around me
That are not of love and light,
That do not bring me joy.
I let go of them right now...
So be it!

Now take three deep breaths and, when exhaling, send the unwanted energy out and away from you.

Window Treatment

Joan loves animals. Dogs and cats are her true companions and friends. She also loves her work, which involves taking care of all the pets in her neighborhood, playing with the cats and walking the dogs, when their owners are away.

One weekend she was looking after a sweet little Maltese named Barbie. Her owner was a grouchy and demanding individual, and his dog was the apple of his eye. Under Joan's care Barbie got sick with persistent diarrhea, and Joan was very worried that Barbie's owner was going to blame her and hold her responsible. She envisioned him yelling at her and being intimidating, and her mind became preoccupied with these images. She was growing more and more distressed as the time of his return grew closer.

She tried the Window Treatment technique, imagining Barbie's owner looking through the window at her, and suddenly her fear of facing him turned into laughter. She repeated the Window

Treatment whenever she noticed her mind becoming preoccupied, and a day later, when the owner returned, she was able to face him without fear. The Window Treatment enabled her to work without the constant anxiety of facing conflict.

HOW TO DO IT

Human interaction can be so fraught with difficulty! At times we feel helplessly exposed to people venting their anger or frustration in unhealthy ways. They may make loud and unreasonable demands, blame, yell, threaten, and throw tantrums. For most of us, this behavior triggers our deep belief systems and we go on autopilot by defending, attacking, or retreating. No matter how we respond, the ingrained views of ourselves that we established in early childhood are the driving force of our inner life and often direct our behavior. Our deep-seated, insecure, and unaware critical voice may say, "She is right; I am no good (not worthy, not deserving)," "If he's looking for a fight, I'll give him one!," and so on. While in some situations your first priority is to make sure that you are safe, in many cases, the Window Treatment is a simple way to defuse the trigger and to soften the bad vibes coming your way.

It may be helpful to consider that this person likely has their own problems that they may be working out from their past; however, you neither have to understand the deeper dynamics of a person's negative behavior nor do you have to accept them.

To relieve your own stress in the moment, draw a window frame around the person's head in your mind's eye and imagine that they are talking through the window of the "Immaturity Ward" of a hospital or that they are a young child assailing you from the window of a nursery school. This may help you to see how silly people's (including our own!) overreactions can be, and it can take the sting out of the situation.

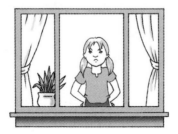

TECHNIQUE 9

Heart Mender Acupressure

Bob was not easily rattled by his emotions. He was a tough guy, and he could keep it together rather well—or so he thought.

At first when his girlfriend broke up with him he felt okay about it, but over the next few days he realized this loss meant more to him than he wanted to admit. He even noticed sadness and tears welling up at the most inopportune moments.

Bob had heard about the beneficial effects of acupressure and was open to this new experience. Massaging the heart mender acupressure point, also called Heart 7, and the heart meridian made him feel calmer. He had to repeat it several times throughout the day, and every time he felt a wave of relaxation that made it easier to cope and go on with his day.

●

Vince, a private in the Army, had decided to visit his family for the Christmas holidays. He was stationed at a base close to the Canadian border and had made the twenty-five-hour journey from his home in south Tennessee to the base on a Greyhound bus a year ago. Vince was now sitting next to me on a plane waiting for takeoff. The twenty-four-year-old had never traveled on an airplane in his life, and his thoughts were racing with anxiety, his heart pounding.

Noticing his agitation, I suggested a way to calm him by pressing on a point along his wrist. After a minute or so of applying pressure with my thumb on the heart mender acupressure point, Vince looked at me with astonishment: he had noticed his heart rate returning to normal and his anxiety lessening. Vince was able to relax and enjoy his first flight.

HOW TO DO IT

Pushing on this acupressure point can help you overcome heartache and emotional distress. Use your thumb to massage Heart 7, located on the inside of both wrists, on the side of your little finger. For some extra help, start on the inside of your palm just under your pinkie finger and massage downward toward and along your wrist, then down your forearm all the way to your funny bone on your elbow. Make sure you stay on the side of your little finger, the inside, also called the "medial" aspect of your palm and arm. You will find tender spots. Massage these a while longer, and you may notice a sense of calm.

HEART MENDER ACUPRESSURE POINT

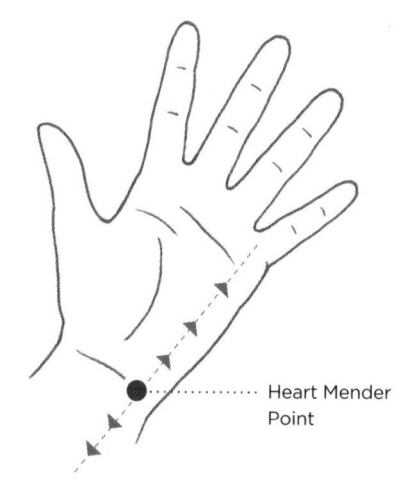

Heart Mender
Point

TECHNIQUE 10

The Happy Traveler

The impact of the economic downturn with its layoffs and spending cuts had created a big change in Abdul's life and that of his family. Abdul was a psychologist and had been working as a consultant for various agencies. He had held steady jobs for many years.

Now he could only find short-term contracts. Interviews for longer-term positions were hard to come by, and the number of competing applicants was higher than ever before. Weighed down by constant stress and fear, as well as worry about the financial well-being of his family, Abdul experienced many sleepless nights filled with churning thoughts. His family life was affected, and his children suffered from his short fuse.

Abdul found that getting a short break from these continuous worries—a holiday for the mind—by using the Happy Traveler technique was very helpful in decreasing his stress level.

•

Glenda had had a difficult year with her health. Physically very active and mentally sharp, she seemed much younger than her eighty-seven years. Over a one-year span she endured five hip surgeries. When she was getting ready for a surgery, her thoughts would wander to one of her favorite locations, a beautiful view overlooking the water at her daughter's cottage. This practice helped her calm her mind and made her body feel more relaxed and peaceful, which in turn helped her recovery process.

·

Like Abdul, you will discover that finding a few minutes of solace using this technique will little by little, with repetition, benefit your mind and body.

HOW TO DO IT

Find a comfortable position sitting or lying down. Close your eyes and put one hand on your heart. Think of a particularly happy moment in your life. Maybe it was a beautiful walk in nature; spending time with family, friends, or pets; an especially enjoyable holiday; the birth of a child; or another special event in your life. Go deeper into this memory in your mind: think of what you saw in front of you, the sounds you heard, and the smells you experienced, and feel the lightness in your body and mind at that time. As you immerse yourself in this memory, you may find a smile on your face and a sense of warmth inside you. Remember that while there are difficult moments in life, there are also happy and inspiring ones. Go back to this same memory at least five times today.

HAPPY HEART

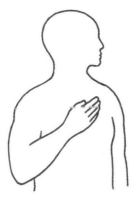

Remembering happy, positive events can normalize your blood pressure and stimulate your brain chemistry. The more time we spend in a happy state of mind, the better we ward off colds and other sickness. The positive effects of this exercise add up over time with more repetition.

This relaxation tool is inspired by the HeartMath modality. You can find more information at www.heartmath.org.

TECHNIQUE 11

Wishing Well

*Problems cannot be solved with the same level
of consciousness that created them.*

—ALBERT EINSTEIN

Of all the exercises in this book, this one is likely both
the easiest and the most difficult!

Most of us can recall having felt betrayed by
someone's behavior, leaving us feeling emotionally
distressed. Perhaps it's a coworker who constantly
undermines you, a family member who does not
include you, a boss who ignores you or sets you up to
fail, or a neighbor who secretly gossips about you.

We all have encountered people in our lives who
have been challenges to us. We may fight back or re-
treat for protection, yet these reactions seldom help us
resolve the situation. Only a radical shift in thinking
will break through these ingrained patterns, and the
only person it can start with is *you*!

It is easy to understand how one can get stuck in patterns of anger and anxiety with negative thoughts focused on the other person. This has been called "stinking thinking" by people in recovery from addictions, as it cuts us off from the creative and positive sides of ourselves and our lives. Such thinking can, over time, suppress our immune system and disrupt the careful balance of hormones and neurotransmitters, causing us to feel truly "off our game" and unhappy. Yet there is another way to deal with negative people that affirms our health and well-being.

HOW TO DO IT

Twice a day, in the morning after waking and just before going to sleep, send some positive thoughts to the person with whom you feel upset. You might simply say in your mind: "I wish you well."

You do not have to love the person, nor do you have to agree with their behavior or forgive them; just go ahead with this technique no matter how much you really mean the thoughts you are sending. With time, the practice will eventually be easier and more meaningful, thus allowing you to live your life in a more peaceful manner. A Buddhist prayer captures this idea nicely:

I wish you well as I wish to be well;
I wish you to be happy as I wish to be happy;
I wish you to be healthy as I wish to be healthy;
I wish you to know peace as I wish to know peace.

If you are really courageous, try doing this throughout your day whenever your thoughts drift back to that person or situation and you feel emotional pain. After some time you will likely notice that your thinking is more positive, releasing you from the unhealthy thoughts and feelings that have been holding you hostage. Take a deep breath and notice how much easier your body-mind feels.

If you can do this, you are indeed a brave person!

TECHNIQUE 12

In a Pinch

OFF AND AWAY WITH ANXIETY

Little Nathan suffered from nightmares. He was three years old, and every night he woke up screaming with terror. His parents were at their wits' end, not knowing how to help him. Due to lack of sleep, everyone felt ragged around the edges.

Nathan's earlobes showed small, sore ridges in the area where the ear attaches to the head. His parents had shown these chronically sore spots to their family doctor who, having no training in ear acupuncture, did not know what to make of them. A good acupuncturist will look for details like this, telltale signs of a problem that may go unnoticed otherwise.

As I mentioned previously, there are acupuncture points on the ear that relate to the entire body and one's emotions. This particular one relates to anxiety, with the right ear expressing conscious fears and the left one unconscious fears. I treated little Nathan with "needle-free acupuncture." After just one treatment, the nightmares vanished.

·

Janice had worked in a family-run business for many years. She was the "assistant for everyone and everything," supporting the owners as best as she could. Over the last few years, her stress level had increased tremendously, with her supervisor becoming more demanding and cantankerous. Even though Janice felt she was doing a good job, it seemed that her boss found flaws with her work no matter how hard she tried. She began searching the job market for a new position, but new employment was very hard to come by. Janice's ear showed dry, rough skin in exactly the same spot as little Nathan's. Treating that area of her earlobe created better mental-emotional balance for Janice.

·

Some days Quinn woke up feeling distressed, with a mix of anxiety and low-grade depression. He found the earlobe pinching and massaging very helpful in calming his emotions, helping him to face the day.

HOW TO DO IT

Using your thumb and index finger, pinch the area where your earlobes meet the side of your head. Roll the skin back and forth or in little circles on both earlobes. Be mindfully vigorous with the massage, feel the good ache, but of course do not press hard enough to cause any bruising. Keep going for one to two minutes or until you feel done. Feel free to repeat this often.

ANXIETY ACUPRESSURE POINT

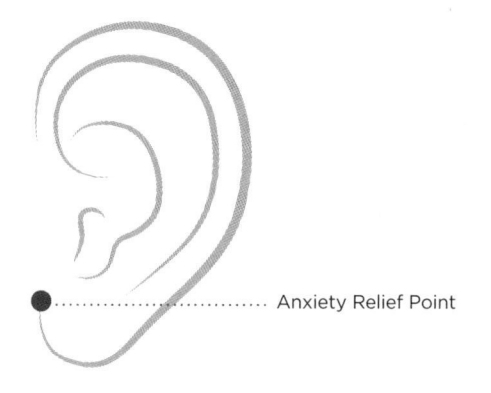

.... Anxiety Relief Point

TECHNIQUE 13

Ocean Sounding Breath

Some mornings Kyle awakes with high levels of anxiety that make him feel unable to get ready for his day. He said, "It feels like very physical anxiety, with my heart racing and my body feeling uneasy, like a vibrating fear." Kyle found the Ocean Sounding Breath technique really helpful; he could feel a "slowing down" all over his body and his heart rate normalizing. He reported, "I also feel an overall calming sensation, and I am always surprised how quickly it improves my sense of well-being."

·

Can you recall a heated argument from your past? Do you remember how your body tightened when you were insulted, felt that you weren't being heard, or perhaps that you were being taken for granted? Our minds often continue to go over and over the argument, the wrongs that have to be righted, and our brilliant brains come up with even better retorts for the next round. Or we may feel crushed by the incident, wanting to withdraw and curl up and hide under the covers. There is a technique that can help you break the vicious circle of stress that arguing with yourself or the people around you can cause. A very calming breathing technique, the Ocean Sounding Breath is named after the soft rushing sound you hear when breathing in this manner.

HOW TO DO IT

Gently tighten the back of your throat as if you want to whisper and slowly, without forcing it, breathe in and out. This will reduce the flow of air going in and out of your lungs. You will hear a sound that reminds you of ocean waves. Now, slowly breathe in and out through your nose, making both the in-breath and the out-breath equally long. You can mindfully count from one to five while you inhale, then count from one to five while you exhale. First, breathe through your nose and fill your belly with air. Once your belly feels full of air, fill your lungs. Exhale in reverse order—let go of the air in your lungs and then in your belly. Start over again and keep going for three minutes or so.

This kind of breathing is used by both yoga and Taoist masters in their meditation practices and can assist in slowing down your thoughts. If you feel distressed while breathing this way, thinking that you are not getting enough air, you are trying too hard. Back off a bit and allow more air to flow into your body.

This way of breathing not only delivers more oxygen to your cells and your brain; it also helps you become more aware of the present moment and your thoughts become more balanced. You may feel a gentle and pleasant tingling in your body, indicating an increased flow of good energy.

Summary of the technique:

1. Gently tighten the back of your throat.

2. Slowly inhale through your nose while counting from one to five. Breathe into your belly first, then into your chest.

3. Slowly exhale through your nose while counting from one to five. Breathe out from your chest first, then your belly.

4. Notice the sound and the calm waves of breath moving in and out of you, filling you with life-giving oxygen and nourishing your brain and body.

Upside Down and Inside Out

*If you want to get a different perspective
on life just tilt your head.*

—ANONYMOUS

This exercise is designed for the physically healthy people among us, the folks who exercise regularly, have a flexible body, and have a healthy circulatory system. If you have any health concerns, please consult your physician before engaging in this posture. This exercise can shift your mental outlook. It also increases the blood supply to your brain, giving it more oxygen.

HOW TO DO IT

Sit comfortably on a chair with your legs wide apart. Slowly lower your upper body, resting your chest on your thighs. Allow your arms to dangle. Keep lowering your head until it hangs upside down between your knees. Do not force it—easy does it! Now, keeping your head down, look around at your surroundings. Do you see an upside-down table, a tree hanging from above, or clouds below the ground? How utterly different the world around you appears when it is upside down! Your surroundings radically shift and the commonplace becomes unfamiliar.

Now, from this perspective, consider the problems that are causing you stress. Do they still have the same impact on you or have they shifted somehow?

Linger in this position as long as feels comfortable, perhaps thirty seconds or so. Now lift your head and upper body very slowly and gently. Do not rush to stand up, but linger a while to reorient yourself. Seeing our world upside down can create a new picture of our lives. Take some time to get a feel for how this experience has changed your outlook.

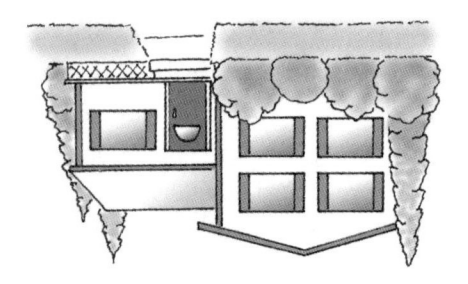

Granny's Words of Wisdom

*That the birds of worry and care fly above your head,
this you cannot change; but that they build nests in
your hair, this you can prevent.*

—CHINESE PROVERB

Recognizing that many of our choices are made out
of fear is a great step toward freedom from a stress-
causing pattern.

Any change to our routine can trigger alertness
and stress inside of us. Whether it is taking on a new
task at work, dealing with a disagreement with a loved
one or friend, needing to have our tires rotated, or
noticing that the grocery store is running out of our
favorite food or our bank account is running low, we
feel our nervous system tighten. Our brain's alarm
system goes on high alert, and we have only a split
second to decide whether to adapt or go into distress,
fear, or anger mode.

Our response, of course, depends to a large extent on our present stress level and our past experiences. We all have been in situations where one simple trigger creates a big response, a knee-jerk reaction: we pull back, engage in anger, or dissolve in tears.

Fortunately there are tools that can help our nervous system quickly recover.

HOW TO DO IT

When you realize that you're having a strong, negative reaction either internally (such as panicky thoughts) or externally (such as harsh words or emotional meltdowns), take a deep breath, look around you, and notice your surroundings. Become aware that everything is in its place. The trees grow where they always have, cars continue to drive by in the same manner, pedestrians head toward their destinations, and birds fly overhead just as before, when life was calmer.

Now pick a wise saying or slogan from the list below that seems fitting for you in this moment; choose intuitively without thinking too hard. Then reflect for a moment about the meaning this slogan has in your life right now. What does it remind you of and how is it helpful to you? You may remember a saying you picked up from your parents, grandparents, or another person instead. Go with that one! What does it mean in your current situation?

Sample Words of Wisdom:

How important is it?

Even after a deep dark night the sun will rise again!

Life goes on.

Expect miracles.

Thy will be done.

I am not in charge.

Live and let live.

Love prevails.

This too shall pass.

Eat the elephant (the insurmountable problem) one bite at a time.

Easy does it.

Let it go.

The Tibetan Smile

GRATITUDE IS THE MOTHER OF SPIRITUAL GROWTH

Phil had not been feeling well. His doctors had given him bad news: he was very ill. His mind was churning, and he felt his muscles tighten with fearful anticipation of his treatment plan. His sympathetic nervous system, which triggers the fight-or-flight response, was in overdrive. Phil knew that only a relaxed body can recover from illness, and he remembered the Tibetan Smile meditation that he had experienced once some time ago. Practicing it daily helped him deal with the stress caused by his illness and contributed to a faster recuperation.

.

Gratitude reconnects us with the positive aspects of our lives. It fosters spiritual growth and gets us out of the trenches of self-pity. Gratitude has been promoted by therapists and spiritual leaders as a healing exercise that connects the mind and spirit. We are usually asked to give thanks to things outside of ourselves, such as our family and friends, shelter and food, or our general safety and well-being.

A beautiful Tibetan prayer asks us to go inward and gratefully acknowledge individual parts of our body-mind. This can boost our immune system, enhance blood supply to the areas we focus on, calm us, and lift our spirits. It can have tremendous health benefits when practiced regularly.

HOW TO DO IT

Get comfortable wherever you are. Take a deep and gentle in-breath, nourishing your body with oxygen. Now gently let go of your breath.

This technique helps you to focus on individual body parts, gratefully acknowledging them when you inhale and sending them a smile of healing when you exhale.

Here is an example:

> *Breathing in I give thanks to my eyes,*
> *breathing out I smile at my eyes.*
>
> *Breathing in I give thanks to my ears,*
> *breathing out I smile at my ears.*

Breathing in I give thanks to my heart,
breathing out I smile at my heart.

Breathing in I give thanks to my brain,
breathing out I smile at my brain.

Breathing in I give thanks to my liver,
breathing out I smile at my liver.

Breathing in I give thanks to my feet,
breathing out I smile at my feet.

While reciting this prayer you may choose to follow a pattern, for example from head to toe, or you may choose to spontaneously follow your inspiration and guide yourself to the organs that come to your awareness. Include the parts of your body that are not entirely healthy at this time. There is no right or wrong way to do this exercise.

TECHNIQUE 17

Exhale

Darius, a twenty-something IT specialist employed by a municipality, was very stressed. His mind was unable to focus, and he felt a heavy weight on his chest. He used to love his job, back when he had a great boss and their working arrangement was built on trust. He now had a different boss who made new rules that restricted him. She tightly controlled his work activity and whereabouts. Darius had lost interest in his work, and his mind was constantly rehashing their unpleasant interactions. Feeling like an orbiting ball of nerves, he had a hard time completing his tasks.

Darius tried the following relaxation exercise, and it helped him settle his mind and relax his body so he could deal more objectively with his new boss.

·

This is a very easy exercise. As with all the other mind-mending techniques, you can do it anywhere and at any time (provided you are not driving a car or operating any heavy machinery, of course!).

HOW TO DO IT

Begin with a mental body scan. Starting with your head and face, notice any tension in the muscles without attaching any judgment to it. Continue doing the same thing as you move down to your neck, arms, chest, abdomen, hips, upper legs, and lower legs, then finally your ankles, feet, and toes. Allow your breath to gently flow in and out of your body as you go.

Now, following the same path you took with your mental body scan, focus on your breathing, paying particular attention to every out-breath. As you gently exhale, let go of muscle tension in each area.

Here is an example:

> *Inhale, then exhale and let go of tension on top of your head;*
>
> *inhale, then exhale and let go of tension in your jaw;*

inhale, then exhale and let go of tension
around your eyes;

and so on.

Keep relaxing every muscle group in your body you can think of, noticing the difference in each area of your body as you release the tension.

Can you imagine the mental and physical energy it required to keep those muscles tightened?

TECHNIQUE 18

Serenity Now!

Whether you have experience with praying or you are a novice at it, there are likely times in your life when you want to reach out to something beyond yourself. The Serenity Prayer has been a comfort to millions of people, including people in recovery from addictions, believers and nonbelievers alike.

HOW TO DO IT

Although this prayer traditionally begins with "God," you may address it to whatever or whomever you like: the "Source," "my Higher Power," "the great Tao," God, Goddess, or simply nature. Pray to no one or to the air around you if that is more comfortable. There are times when writing this prayer on sticky notes and wallpapering my house with it seems like a pretty good idea!

The Serenity Prayer

God, grant me the serenity
to accept the things I cannot change,
courage to change the things I can,
and wisdom to know the difference.

I also like this addition from United Kingdom Codependents Anonymous:

Grant me patience with the changes that
take time,
appreciation of all that I have,
tolerance of those with different struggles,
and the strength to get up and try again,
one day at a time.

Smoke and Mirrors, aka "The Splinter in the Eye"

Some folks are very annoying. I can think of a handful of people who are downright irritating. Not to mention the ones who have poor manners and are out to get me with their words and actions.

—ANONYMOUS

Has your brain ever pushed the repeat and shuffle buttons after encountering behaviors or actions like those mentioned in the quote above? Have such behaviors triggered an emotional reaction in you? Psychologists tell us that our mental-emotional triggers are judgments that we have of ourselves but are not aware of. These self-judgments live in our subconscious, hidden from view, and usually are not true statements about ourselves. Becoming aware of these false belief systems has been called "shadow work," meaning that we "pull" our hidden character traits and beliefs out of the shadows where we cannot see them and bring them to our awareness.

It is like looking in the mirror and seeing your reflection and then realizing that the image you see is not your real body but only a flat, two-dimensional reflection. Your true body is much more complete, beautiful, and full of life and depth. Letting go of negative thoughts and judgments will enable us to live our lives more wholly and peacefully. No longer judging ourselves and others so harshly allows us to be more accepting of ourselves and can magically transform how we see other people as well. Instead of being emotionally reactive and holding others responsible for our thoughts, we are free to see people for who they are and not project our opinions onto them. This is liberating and leaves much more mind-space and energy for our own creativity and joy.

Robert Johnson (the Jungian psychologist, not to be confused with the blues musician with the same name) wrote many books about owning your own shadow. Marion Woodman and Robert Bly are also famous for their books and workshops on how to engage the shadow side of ourselves.

It is curious that the most difficult part of shadow work is not becoming aware of our negative traits and judgments, but becoming aware of our positive traits and talents that we have pushed aside.

Emotional triggers are actually a great gift because they reveal what is hiding in the shadow side of our psyche. Being triggered by someone's behavior does not mean that you are exactly like that person or that you need to forgive or embrace the behavior. It only means that you can disagree without your blood pressure and heart rate rising and your immune system weakening. It means that your own mental energy has more time and space for positive engagement, which will enhance your life, your creativity, and your soul's journey.

I am compelled to give you a word of caution as well: judging others for negative and challenging behavior does not imply that you have to put up with any form of abuse—verbal, psychological, or physical—and tell yourself that all you need to do is process it and you will be fine and released from your difficulties. Abuse is not tolerable, and a skilled therapist can help you gain more clarity in your situation and assist you in finding the right path to healing.

HOW TO DO IT

You need the following items:

1. A generous dose of self-honesty

2. A pen

3. A piece of lined paper (or, use the blank lined page provided after this exercise)

Divide your piece of paper into two columns. On the left side, write down your grievances with a particular person or situation. Take one line for every item, writing down what you do not like or what triggers you. On the right side, across from each entry on the left side, write whether you have ever behaved in a similar way (see example on page 77).

This list is not about you feeling guilty for your actions, nor does it mean that you now agree with the person's behavior or the situation. You may just have the smallest seed of these tendencies in yourself that triggered your emotions. Rather, this list is intended to serve as a reminder that we are all human, that all of us are trapped in behavior patterns and modes of thinking that are not always compassionate or positive. Dealing with our triggers can help us feel calmer, even when a situation is disagreeable. We just do not have to keep replaying these old tapes, and we can release parts of our shadow and reduce resentments that only hurt us.

When we are triggered, we are revealing to ourselves that we have a faulty belief system about ourselves. Sometime in our past, maybe when we were young and impressionable, we subscribed to deep beliefs about ourselves that most likely are not true at all. Becoming aware of this will help fix the automatic program running in our subconscious.

The more frequently you do this exercise, the more you will notice changes in your thinking. Remember that what other people do or say has nothing to do with you, only with them and their state of mind. As my mentor Ruth liked to say, "What other people think of me is their problem." You will very likely be more convinced of the correctness of that attitude when you have completed this exercise.

Here is an example:

She did not greet me.	I remember not greeting my sister-in-law at the family reunion.
He always interrupts me.	I remember that my friend complained about me interrupting her.
She gossips.	I have talked about others at times.
He is a bully.	I have dominated my children at times.
She is so miserly.	I have refused to give money to relatives who needed it.

My List

TECHNIQUE 20

Decisions, Decisions

Making a decision can be agonizing! Having to decide what to do with our free time, what to eat, whether to drastically change our life by moving, taking a new job, ending a relationship, or going through with a particular medical treatment can use up a lot of our precious energy and consume our thoughts. Making decisions when there is much at stake can be especially stressful.

Our minds become so preoccupied that we are oblivious to the present moment, not engaging with ourselves and our surroundings. We may feel exhausted and even experience short-term memory problems.

Some of us are apt to arrive at a decision too swiftly, whereas others have a habit of weighing the options until the last train has left the station. The ability to make decisions may be influenced by our genetic makeup and is also affected by our environment. At times low thyroid function or a brain "disorganized" by allergies, drugs, or environmental sensitivities can affect our ability to be decisive.

Sometimes when faced with making a decision, we may be stuck thinking that there are only two choices, when it often turns out that there are other possibilities. A little brainstorming may help you realize there are many more options than just a "yes" or "no."

Being preoccupied with decision making eats up large chunks of our energy, and many clients have consulted me for the sole purpose of getting help with making choices. You've probably noticed that as soon as you make up your mind, you feel as if a weight has been lifted off your shoulders, leaving you free and energized to move on with life.

The best decisions come from the heart. Our Western society has placed much importance on our higher thinking and reasoning faculties, and there is no doubt that gathering detailed information about an issue to be decided upon can be useful in making a good choice. But once the "think tank" has been filled to satisfaction with crucial information, it is time to turn our attention away from the brain and sink into our hearts and "guts" to help make a decision.

HOW TO DO IT

1. Make sure you understand the implications of your decision and that you have sufficient information regarding your choices.

2. Pick one of the other techniques in this book, such as Square Breathing or Ocean Sounding Breath, to help ground and center your thoughts and body.

3. Now put your hand on your heart and close your eyes.

4. Go through each possible solution in your mind, one at a time, each time paying attention to your body.

As you consider each solution, does your body feel good, happy, uplifted, or at ease? This is a clear indication to pick this choice. Or is there a sense of uncertainty, restriction, or a lowering of your spirits or physical energy level? This would indicate a clear "no," or at least suggest that you shouldn't rush into that particular action. Your body is clearly trying to tell you something when it feels uneasy. It means that a particular choice is not the right one.

There may be a concern that we will pick the easiest solution using this method, but once you are familiar with this process you will notice that your authentic body-mind never chooses the easy way out. You will be more likely to make choices that enhance your life and complete your "soul journey" at some level, even if it creates more effort, work, or some inconvenience. A decision made by listening to your body can propel you forward in your life and enrich your experience of being human. That is the beauty of living from your heart.

HEAD, HEART, GUT

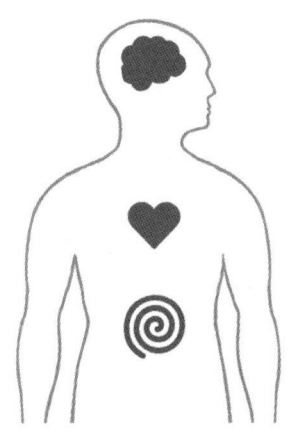

Part II:

Theory and Background on the Techniques

The Mind-Body Connection

The Western world has struggled with the relationship between mind and body since the age of reason. Many people are not even aware that the relationship is debated and don't know whether the mind does interact with the body. However, modern research is fascinated by the connection and interaction between the mind and the body, and a growing number of people are starting to see what healers the world over, especially the Chinese and other Asian and native cultures, have known for centuries: that mind and body are intimately entwined. Even though most Western doctors still treat the body and mind as if they are separate systems, recent scientific evidence shows that they are very closely interrelated and have a very tight network of communication, a two-way connection, functioning somewhat like a walkie-talkie. Nothing happens in the body without the mind quickly noticing and responding to the information received—and vice versa.

Imagine two pieces of duct tape stuck together on their sticky sides. They are nearly impossible to pull apart. When you tug on one piece, the other responds by moving along with it and not giving way. That is exactly how closely our body and mind are connected. Without us being consciously aware of it, our mind is constantly busy receiving sensory data and other input. For example, we know that 90 percent of our human communication is nonverbal, and the brain and body are able to interpret these signals, oblivious to our conscious mind. That includes listening to what someone says and subconsciously understanding whether that person's tone of voice, stance, and facial expression do or do not match what is said. If the words spoken do not match the nonverbal cues, it causes confusion and discomfort.

Our subconscious takes in the nonverbal cues like a watch dog, informs our glands and organs of this input, and sets off a cascade of reactions in our body, either perking up our immune system and sense of well-being or causing distress, depending on the type of experience. Persistent unresolved, negative, or confusing communication, especially from the important people in our lives, causes negative emotions that can eventually weaken our immune system, making us more vulnerable to illness. Fear of an immediate threat engages our adrenal glands, which secrete hormones that increase our endurance and prepare us to face that threat—but only temporarily! In the long-term, stress overload from physical or emotional threats results in depleted adrenal gland function, which in turn leads to daytime fatigue, insomnia, exhaustion, and difficulty coping.

Scientist Candace Pert's life work revolved around proving that our mind influences the state of hormonal well-being in our body and showed that positive experiences give us a sense of well-being and strengthen our immune system. In his book *Biology of Belief,* scientist and researcher Dr. Bruce Lipton eloquently describes how our thoughts and emotions influence the expression of our genetic code. Indeed, the earlier model of genes as being parts of a fixed and complete system that are activated like light switches at birth has given rise to a much more plastic model in recent years. We have come to understand that our life experience, our nutrition, and our mind-set will influence whether our genetic code will turn on certain genes or leave them dormant.

Medical research has also shown us that life-threatening illnesses frequently occur after high levels of stress-causing events, such as the loss of a job or a loved one, a divorce, or other major psychological trauma. In fact, even joyous events, such as getting married or having a child and the adjustments these major life changes require, may signal a stress response that can cause health issues.

Fortunately, we now have a better understanding of these mind-body dynamics, which allows us to make a more conscious connection between our bodies and minds and create a more holistic experience that promotes both physical and emotional health. This, in turn, switches on the immune system and balances the healthy expression of our genetic code. In other words, the happier, more inspired, and creative you are, the better you can cope with stressful situations, and the more you are able to process stressful events, the healthier you will be.

Yes, I know, our grandparents talked about the importance of positive thinking a long time ago—and now we have scientific proof of their wisdom!

•

The Mechanics of Acupressure and the Meridian System

Acupressure and acupuncture make use of the body's meridian system, which was discovered a few thousand years ago by Chinese physicians. The meridian system is akin to the nervous system, but it is separate from the anatomical structures that we know in Western medicine.

Imagine twelve long, narrow "rivers" of energy flowing through either side of your body along prescribed paths. They are symmetrical, meaning they flow on each side of your body from head to toe and fingers, and vice versa. These rivers, or channels of energy, are important to our health in how they relate to our organs, other body parts, moods, and emotions.

We know that these channels, with about as many acupuncture points sprinkled on them as there are days in the year, carry an electrical charge that we can measure with an "ohmmeter," a device electricians use to measure electrical resistance. An acupuncture point conducts more electricity than its surrounding skin, and applying pressure to the point will help to balance this flow of electrical energy and create a self-healing response in your body.

Diagnosis in Chinese Medicine

In ancient China, autopsies were forbidden and medicine became the subtle art of "listening" to the body-mind. Chinese doctors were trained to be very observant and fine-tuned in the art of assessing their patients. There are three major ways that specialists of Chinese medicine find out what is going on in the body; namely taking a careful history, taking the pulse in a way unique to this discipline, and looking at the tongue.

The first method is obvious and is used in any type of medicine. The patient reports as exactly as possible what he or she experiences in the body and mind; the aches and pains; and particular circumstances, patterns, and time frames of the complaints. The second method, taking the pulse, is a way of discovering what is going on inside the body by taking several pulses on both wrists. Chinese pulse diagnosis offers a window into the function of organ systems without blood work, lab tests, and imaging. It takes many years of practice and learning to perfect the art and interpretation of "pulse diagnosis."

A number of years ago I traveled to China to study medical Qigong, an ancient system of postures, movements, and meditation techniques to create mind-body harmony. We visited a traditional Chinese medicine hospital and underwent Chinese pulse diagnosis performed by doctors on staff. The diagnosis established by these doctors who knew nothing about our medical history was astounding. They accurately described symptoms, imbalances, and illnesses in many of us.

When I learned the art of Chinese medicine at a course in Toronto, our teacher had us practice pulse diagnosis on other students. As I was feeling the pulse position relating to the heart, I noticed a "weak" pulse wave under the tip of my finger. The student, an upper-middle-aged man, confirmed that he had had a heart attack a couple of years previously. It seemed almost eerie to me then, but this kind of experience has become commonplace to me now after practicing Chinese medicine for more than two decades.

In addition to history taking and pulse diagnosis, Chinese medicine specialists practice the art of tongue diagnosis. The color, shape, and size of the tongue reveal much about a person's state of health and the condition of his or her specific meridians.

These three diagnostic tools give the doctors the information required to assess the meridian system and treat their patients. It is an eye-opening experience to have a doctor who is well trained in Chinese medicine and pulse diagnosis tell you about your state of health on a mental, emotional, and physical level without even knowing your name or your health history.

•

Famous Canadian neurophysiologist Dr. Bruce Pomeranz has conducted extensive research on how acupuncture affects the meridian system and found that potent neurotransmitters are released that benefit the body's healing system. This research is very important and meaningful; it does not, however, explain exactly why stimulating very specific acupressure points can help certain illnesses and support the health of an individual. Therefore, if you decide that you would like to explore using acupuncture or acu-pressure to treat a specific condition beyond the tech-niques in this book, finding a well-trained practitioner will make all the difference.

*

The Man in the Ear: Ear Acupuncture

Not all acupuncture is Chinese. It took a passionate and observant French physician by the name of Paul Nogier to discover the power of acupuncture points of the ear. You may have heard of foot reflexology, a system involving pressure points on the foot that reflect different parts of the body. It turns out that the ears, like the feet, are "reflex organs." The story of ear acupuncture reads a bit like a fairy tale, albeit a true one, and when I first read about it as a sixteen-year-old, I was fascinated, as I still am many decades later.

Here is the abbreviated story:

Dr. Paul Nogier was a French general practitioner with a highly inquisitive nature. The intricate expressions and hidden physiology of the body fascinated him. He discovered that massaging certain points on the ears of his patients drastically reduced their back pain. At times he had to massage the ear quite hard, which, as you can imagine, could be rather painful. His patients, however, were thrilled because the ear massage often alleviated long-standing back pain.

Nogier then started to use acupuncture needles on those specific points in the ear, a method that gave a gentler stimulation of the "back pain points" with good results.

The story does not end there. One day while he was holding the pulse of a patient, he touched certain "active" points on the ear and felt the patient's pulse shift under his thumb. It felt stronger or weaker in certain spots. He discovered that when there is a dysfunction or problem in a particular body part or organ, specific points on the ear are tender to the touch and, when stimulated, also shift the person's pulse wave. That was the birth of auricular medicine, by now a very sophisticated and refined modality practiced by medical doctors and practitioners around the globe.

What makes a point tender or "active"? Acupuncture points in the ear become active or tender when there is a problem in the body or mind. Active points carry a stronger electrical charge than the surrounding skin. The conductivity of electricity is higher in an active acupuncture point in the ear compared to the surrounding area, as shown using an ohmmeter. So whether you have back pain, are anxious or depressed, or have a sore tooth, your ear acupuncture expert can find certain points that have more electrical current flow across the skin in contrast to the surrounding area and that, when treated, can help you feel better. Auricular medicine has developed further into a sophisticated method for finding and adjusting underlying causes of health issues. It is particularly helpful for chronic illness.

·

The Benefits of Upside Down

Upside-down positions have been practiced by yogis and yoginis for centuries. There are at least two benefits to hanging your head upside down, or "inversion," as it is called in yoga. I briefly mentioned the first one in Technique 14: Upside Down, Inside Out: it allows us to change the perception of the world we are used to. In our everyday life, the earth is beneath us and the heavens are above, we walk on our legs and feet, cars drive on top of the roads, and birds fly above us. We are so used to this view that we do not challenge it; we do not question why things are the way they are.

Often when we can't untangle a mental-emotional issue, we are stuck in a certain gear. We can't move on or find a solution because our thinking repeatedly follows certain tracks in our brain, moving along the same nerve pathways and turning them into ruts. In order to unstick our thinking, it is very helpful to change our perception. Doing so can dislodge our habits of thinking so we use new nerve pathways and are able to find new views and solutions to a problem.

The perception of seeing the earth above us, hanging over the sky, trees growing upside down, water glasses suspended upside down without spilling, and folks around us standing on their heads jolts our understanding and frees up our brains. The very same thing happens with the problems we are facing. Suddenly more options open up before our very eyes, and we can see a variety of solutions that were unavailable to our previous, more limited thinking patterns.

There are also biological advantages to the physical act of placing our head lower than our feet. Inverting our head allows gravity to increase the blood supply to our brain, providing good oxygen and nutrients. Also, our brain not only consists of the nerves folded into white and gray matter that most of us are familiar with; it also houses two very important glands, the pineal and pituitary glands (think of them as hormone factories) as well as higher control towers (the thalamus and hypothalamus, for example). The pineal gland is very important for our life rhythms, sleep and aging. In esoteric traditions, this gland is thought to be the seat of higher consciousness, our connection to the spirit within, or God. When we are anxious or depressed, we are disconnected from our inner being. Increasing the blood flow to and improving lymphatic drainage from the important glands in our brain helps with nourishment and detoxification, and *voila!*—the brain functions much better!

Our pituitary gland has the big task of keeping most of the other glands in our body stimulated and regulated. It regulates the thyroid gland and the adrenals and is important in maintaining blood pressure and producing oxytocin, the "feel good" hormone that helps us physically and socially bond with people. Oxytocin is also known to cause contractions during childbirth and is released during intimacy, making us feel close to our romantic partner.

The pituitary gland sits in a small, protected, bony cave in the brain that opens and drains at the top. Imagine a glass of water: you can empty it by drinking it with a straw, or you can turn it upside down and the water will flow much more freely. This is similar to what happens with the hormones of the pituitary gland. No worries, though—you will not dump out too much of the good hormones at a time, as your body is too smart for that. Gravity will, however, improve the circulation of the hormones, provide more blood supply and drainage, clear more lymph, and tune up the gland's function.

You can see that inverting your head may help those good hormones go where they need to go: to their target glands and organs. This is another reason why inverting our body for a while will make us happier!

•

The Workings of the Ocean
Sounding Breath

The Ocean Sounding Breath is another ancient yogic technique of great benefit to our Western lifestyle.

We all know that breathing comes naturally, without any effort from our conscious mind. Thank goodness we don't have to constantly remind ourselves to take a breath! Breathing is one of our body's automatic functions, along with our heart beating and the digestion of our food. No conscious effort is required to fill our lungs and rhythmically pump our heart because the autonomic nervous system picks up clues and cues from our surroundings to modify the automatic activities going on inside of us.

The quality of our breathing is influenced by our deeper states of mind, and when we become anxious, stressed, and preoccupied, our breathing has a tendency to suffer by becoming shallower. Without being consciously aware of it, we may even take long breaks in between our in-breaths and out-breaths, thus further reducing the intake of life-giving oxygen.

Our autonomic nervous system, also called our involuntary nervous system, is crucial in influencing many of the automatic activities of our bodies. There are two branches that pull this internal function in different directions, like the ends of a teeter-totter. The one branch, the sympathetic nervous system, can enable us to quickly burst into a thousand-yard sprint, running away from perceived danger, whereas the opposing branch, the parasympathetic nervous system, can help us relax, digest, heal, and turn on our immune system. Both systems are very important, as we need to be able to fight or flee (sympathetic) or heal and relax (parasympathetic) to maintain our bodies.

Anxiety leads to a state of stress, causing our fight-or-flight mechanism to run in high gear. Modern-day stress and anxiety rarely prompt us to actually fight or flee, but they leave our internal systems revved up at high speed as though we needed to. This, of course, results in high levels of distress to our bodies, leading to a multitude of illnesses.

While we do not have control over our autonomic nervous system, we can influence it indirectly by making sure we exercise, relax, and restore ourselves through activities—or, rather, non-activities—such as gazing at the clouds, listening to music, laughing and visiting with people we love, painting a picture, watching old movies, or practicing the techniques in this book.

Breathing more deeply and deliberately can help our entire system to slow down, engaging the heal and relax system (parasympathetic) and increasing our oxygen intake. It can revive us, make us feel more alive, clear our thoughts, and energize us.

Paying more attention to our breathing cycle by slowing down our breath and being more mindful and conscious can have a calming effect on our mind by distracting us from its spinning and revolving thoughts. By practicing the simple Ocean Sounding Breath technique, we derive all the benefits of meditation.

Ancient yogis also spoke of the positive effects of the Ocean Sounding Breath on our intestines because it causes our diaphragm, the breathing muscle, to contract more fully, thus gently massaging the insides of our abdomen. This improves blood flow, lymph drainage, nutrient uptake, and detoxification.

I have never encountered anyone who did not notice some calming after only a few minutes of practicing the Ocean Sounding Breath.

•

The BodyTalk System Explained:
BodyTalk Cortices

BodyTalk and BodyTalk Access are energy medicine modalities developed by Dr. John Veltheim, an Australian chiropractor, acupuncturist, Reiki master, and philosopher.

BodyTalk is a very gentle yet profound way of balancing, aligning, and synchronizing one's body and its functions, thus improving the body's ability to heal itself. A powerful modality that can be learned by anyone, it is largely based on two concepts:

1. The body becomes "dysfunctional" when communication within or among organs, body parts, or the brain/mind becomes impaired. By finding the areas that need to improve and balancing their communication, the body can heal itself on its own.

2. The innate intelligence of the body knows exactly how it needs to address its healing and which problems should take priority. This

means we can use BodyTalk techniques to balance and enhance the body's systems by tapping into the body's deeper wisdom. A practitioner uses neuro-muscular feedback as a tool to establish the type and sequence of balances used for each individual.

Any form of assault on the body, be it emotional, viral, or a physical injury, can potentially break down the sophisticated communication process in the body. Our bodies function as systems. The liver alone is responsible for five hundred chemical reactions, so it makes sense that it takes a good communication system to streamline the functions of the liver, let alone the entire body. Just as a factory production line would break down without a proper communication plan, so would the function of the body break down without constant communication within and among all its parts.

To understand this concept a little better, imagine going to a classical music concert. When you arrive early at the concert hall, you hear the musicians tune their instruments in the orchestra pit, and it sounds disjointed and inharmonious. During the performance, however, you hear beautiful music with the help of the conductor and musicians listening to one another and reading their sheet music. This is similar to what happens in the physiology of our bodies as communication among the various parts helps achieve harmony and balance.

The BodyTalk Cortices technique is a stand-alone application of BodyTalk and BodyTalk Access modalities. The hands are used as a focusing tool to connect the two hemispheres of the brain. By opening up the connections between the hemispheres—the highways and country roads, so to speak—the brain becomes unblocked, better able to function, and capable of paying attention to its needs. This opening of brain pathways allows for processing of thoughts, emotions, and other healthy brain functions.

For information about courses on this topic offered all over the world, visit the website of the BodyTalk Association: www.bodytalksystem.com.

•

Resources

Websites

Heartmath Institute:
  www.heartmath.org

International BodyTalk Association:
  www.bodytalksystem.com

Books

Gach, Michael Reed. *Acupressure's Potent Points.*
New York: Bantam, 1990.

Grabhorn, Lynn. *Excuse Me, Your Life Is Waiting:
The Astonishing Power of Feelings.* Newburyport, MA:
Hampton Roads Publishing Company, 2000.

Johnson, Robert. *Owning Your Own Shadow:
Understanding the Dark Side of the Psyche.* San
Francisco: Harper Collins, 1991.

Lipton, Bruce H. *The Biology of Belief: Unleashing the
Power of Consciousness, Matter and Miracles.* Rev. ed.
Carlsbad, CA: Hay House, 2008.

Pert, Candace. *Molecules of Emotion: The Science
behind Mind-Body Medicine.* New York: Simon and
Schuster, 1999.

Acknowledgments

I am grateful to the fabulous editorial and production team at Hazelden Publishing for their contributions and for giving me the opportunity to make these techniques available to more people. Thanks also to Linda Roghaar for her expertise and to my friends and clients for their valuable contributions, with a special thank-you to MeeNah Pelland.

About the Author

Katrin Schubert has dedicated her career to helping her fellow human beings heal their bodies, minds, and spirits with natural medicine. After completing her medical degree and a PhD in 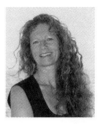 human genetics at the University of Hamburg, and receiving international training in England, the Czech Republic, India, China, Canada, and the United States, she opened her holistic health clinics in Kingston and Gananoque, Ontario, Canada. Katrin also has a science degree from Queen's University in Kingston. You can contact Katrin through her website: www.drkatrin.com.

About Hazelden Publishing

As part of the Hazelden Betty Ford Foundation, Hazelden Publishing offers both cutting-edge educational resources and inspirational books. Our print and digital works help guide individuals in treatment and recovery, and their loved ones. Professionals who work to prevent and treat addiction also turn to Hazelden Publishing for evidence-based curricula, digital content solutions, and videos for use in schools, treatment programs, correctional programs, and electronic health records systems. We also offer training for implementation of our curricula.

Through published and digital works, Hazelden Publishing extends the reach of healing and hope to individuals, families, and communities affected by addiction and related issues

For more information about Hazelden publications,
please call **800-328-9000**
or visit us online at **hazelden.org/bookstore**.

Other Titles That May Interest You

How to Change Your Thinking

Hazelden Quick Guides

This collection of four eBooks applies the proven methods of Rational Emotive Behavior Therapy to challenge the irrational thoughts and beliefs that contribute to the debilitating effects of shame, anger, depression, and anxiety.

How to Change Your Thinking about Shame
Order no. EB4804

How to Change Your Thinking about Anger
Order no. EB4802

How to Change Your Thinking about Depression
Order no. EB4803

How to Change Your Thinking about Anxiety
Order no. EB4805

Almost Anxious

Is My (or My Loved One's) Worry or Distress a Problem?
Luana Marques, PhD, with Eric Metcalf, MPH

In *Almost Anxious,* Luana Marques, PhD, describes the spectrum of anxiety symptoms, from normal situational anxiety on one end to a full-blown diagnosable anxiety disorder on the other.
Order no. 4388; eBook EB4388

For more information or to order these or other resources from Hazelden Publishing, call **800-328-9000** or visit **hazelden.org/bookstore.**